Cambridge Elements

Elements of Improving Quality and Safety in Healthcare
edited by
Mary Dixon-Woods,* Katrina Brown,* Sonja Marjanovic,†
Tom Ling,† Ellen Perry,* Graham Martin*, Gemma Petley*,
and Claire Dipple*
*THIS Institute (The Healthcare Improvement Studies Institute)
†RAND Europe

HUMAN FACTORS AND ERGONOMICS

Mark Sujan[1] and Laura Pickup[2]
[1]*University of York*
[2]*LP Human Factors*

THIS.Institute The Healthcare Improvement Studies Institute

The Health Foundation

CAMBRIDGE UNIVERSITY PRESS

CAMBRIDGE
UNIVERSITY PRESS

Shaftesbury Road, Cambridge CB2 8EA, United Kingdom

One Liberty Plaza, 20th Floor, New York, NY 10006, USA

477 Williamstown Road, Port Melbourne, VIC 3207, Australia

314–321, 3rd Floor, Plot 3, Splendor Forum, Jasola District Centre, New Delhi – 110025, India

Cambridge University Press is part of Cambridge University Press & Assessment, a department of the University of Cambridge.

We share the University's mission to contribute to society through the pursuit of education, learning and research at the highest international levels of excellence.

www.cambridge.org
Information on this title: www.cambridge.org/9781047756013

DOI: 10.1017/9781047755993

First published 2026

A catalogue record for this publication is available from the British Library

A Cataloging-in-Publication data record for this Element is available from the Library of Congress

ISBN 978-1-047-75601-3 Paperback
ISSN 2754-2912 (online)
ISSN 2754-2904 (print)

Human Factors and Ergonomics

Elements of Improving Quality and Safety in Healthcare

DOI: 10.1017/9781047755993
First published online: June 2026

Mark Sujan[1] and Laura Pickup[2]
[1]University of York
[2]LP Human Factors

Author for correspondence: Mark Sujan, mark.sujan@york.ac.uk

Abstract: Human Factors and Ergonomics (HFE) is a discipline concerned with designing interactions in sociotechnical systems to improve both system performance and human well-being. This Element introduces the core principles of HFE, tracing its development from multidisciplinary efforts to solve practical problems in military operations during the Second World War to its current application in healthcare improvement. The Element acknowledges the growing role of HFE in areas such as the design of the physical environment, medical device design, learning from patient safety incidents, and safety investigations. A critical reflection highlights persistent challenges, including conceptual ambiguity, structural and practical barriers to HFE integration, and the need for both a stronger evidence base and a compelling business case. The Element concludes by identifying future priorities for advancing HFE in healthcare, including continuing professional development and career pathways, embedding HFE in regulation and policy, and adopting evaluation approaches suited to complex systems. This title is also available as open access on Cambridge Core.

Keywords: human factors, ergonomics, systems thinking, patient safety, sociotechnical systems

ISBNs: 9781047756013 (PB), 9781047755993 (OC)
ISSNs: 2754-2912 (online), 2754-2904 (print)

Contents

1 Introduction

Human Factors and Ergonomics (HFE) is about designing work systems that support people and enhance both system performance and human well-being. The International Ergonomics Association (IEA) defines HFE as 'the scientific discipline concerned with the understanding of interactions among humans and other elements of a system, and the profession that applies theory, principles, data, and methods to design in order to optimise human well-being and overall system performance'.[1]

Three features of this definition can be highlighted.

(1) HFE is based on a systems approach. This recognises that outcomes in complex settings like healthcare rarely stem from a single cause, but instead emerge from the dynamic interactions between people, tasks, technologies, physical spaces, organisational structures, and wider regulatory, socioeconomic, and political environments.[2] Accordingly, HFE provides a scientific foundation for understanding how these interactions shape work and produce outcomes.
(2) HFE is a profession that is practice-oriented, seeking to apply foundational knowledge to the design of work systems.
(3) HFE seeks to influence a broad range of outcomes, including safety, efficiency, usability, and well-being.

Although HFE originated in military, aviation, and industrial settings, its core concerns – issues such as system design, workflows, the design of work environments, and human well-being – are now increasingly recognised as important to healthcare. However, despite growing interest, HFE remains only partially understood in healthcare, where it is often narrowly associated with teamwork or aviation-style training,[3] and its practical application may be misunderstood or misrepresented.[4] HFE is not about finding 'the human factor' as the cause of accidents, nor is it limited to individual performance or 'non-technical skills'.

To show how HFE has evolved into the discipline and practice it is today, Section 2 outlines its historical development and introduces key models and methods that have shaped the field. Section 3 then presents examples of how HFE thinking has been applied in healthcare. Section 4 provides a critical reflection on the current status of HFE in healthcare, including its limitations and potential, while Section 5 offers an outlook on future directions for the field.

2 What Do We Mean by Human Factors and Ergonomics?

The IEA definition, adopted in 2000, provides a strong description of HFE, but several other definitions exist. Almost from the outset, there has been considerable debate about what HFE stands for and how it should be defined. This debate continues as new problems emerge and as the discipline – and its scholars and practitioners – continue to adapt, reflect, and redefine their roles.

To clarify what HFE can offer, it is helpful to look briefly at its evolution from its origins during the wartime period of the early 1940s, before turning to its application in healthcare and some of the main models and methods used in this domain.

2.1 The Origins of Human Factors and Ergonomics

The discipline of HFE emerged from practical military problems experienced during the Second World War.[5] During this period, people had to manage more extreme environments and increasingly complex technologies and communication systems. Numerous incidents were attributed to human error, most notably in military aviation, where several aircraft crashed as pilots were struggling with fatigue, lack of adequate oxygen supply, and poorly designed cockpit layouts.

A well-known early example of HFE design thinking is the work of Paul Fitts and Alphonse Chapanis on B-17 and B-25 landing accidents. Pilots were mistakenly retracting the landing gear instead of lowering the flaps – initially labelled 'pilot error'. Fitts and Chapanis interviewed pilots and examined the cockpit. They recognised that the two controls were identical in shape and placed side by side, making confusion likely under stress. Their simple redesign using shape coding, in this instance a wheel-shaped knob for the gear and a wing-shaped one for the flaps, eliminated these errors almost immediately, reframing 'human error' as a design problem.

Patrick Waterson describes the history of HFE in the UK by chronicling the development of the Ergonomics Research Society (ERS), now the Chartered Institute of Ergonomics and Human Factors.[6–8] As in the US, several research institutes in the UK supported wartime efforts through improved design of equipment and controls. These include, for example, the Royal Air Force Physiological Laboratory (later the Institute of Aviation Medicine), the Cambridge Psychological Laboratory, the Medical Research Council Applied Psychology Unit, and the School of Anatomy at Oxford University. Their work on issues such as pilot fatigue and pilot error, radar operator effectiveness, and visual perception under stress led to improvements in control layouts, anatomically appropriate seat design for combat, and protective equipment.

The term 'ergonomics' is usually credited to Hywel Murrell, a psychologist at the Admiralty Naval Motion Study Unit. In 1949, Murrell convened a meeting of like-minded individuals to discuss the formation of a forum to exchange ideas and expertise between the disciplines that had contributed to enhanced human performance during the wartime period. Initially, these disciplines were anatomy, physiology, and psychology. The meeting led to the adoption of the term 'ergonomics' and the establishment of the ERS as a formal community through which to develop foundational knowledge.

From the outset, it was challenging to define exactly what ergonomics was, and debate within the ERS and the wider ergonomics community about the scope of the discipline has persisted. Over the decades, the HFE community has had to adapt to technological and societal change in order to remain relevant. The wartime focus on relatively clearly defined, often manual, tasks shifted considerably during the 1960s with large-scale automation, and then again during the 1970s with the rise of business and office computing technologies. Issues of industrial ergonomics and safety-critical systems – such as nuclear power plant control room design – became increasingly important. This was accompanied by a move towards cognitive ergonomics and the notion of joint cognitive systems and cognitive systems engineering, i.e. the consideration of how people and computing technologies work together to carry out cognitive functions, with cognition distributed across people, tools, and environments.[9] Major accidents, such as the 1986 Chernobyl disaster, further broadened the scope to include (safety) cultures and organisational structures.[10,11]

HFE has always been multidisciplinary, drawing on fields such as anatomy, physiology, and psychology, and later industrial design, systems engineering, computer science, cognitive science, organisational sociology, and public health. Over time, specialisms – such as human–computer interaction and user experience design – have emerged, making it hard to draw clearly defined boundaries around HFE.

In its early years, HFE and the ERS in the UK were regarded primarily as an academic field and a forum for bringing together different disciplines, rather than as a professional practice. Over time, tensions emerged between these multidisciplinary roots and the growing need for consistent, applied professional work. These tensions helped drive the development of HFE as a defined profession. In 1977, the ERS reflected this shift by changing its name to the Ergonomics Society, dropping the explicit focus on research. In 2009, the name changed again, this time to the Institute of Ergonomics and Human Factors, in part to reflect international usage of the term 'human factors'. In 2014, the institute was awarded a royal charter and became the Chartered Institute of Ergonomics and Human Factors. Today, around 600 chartered ergonomists are registered.

This institutional development reflects a broader maturation of the field, from a multidisciplinary forum towards a defined profession with a shared set of principles and practices. While the debate continues about the scope of HFE and the relationship between foundational research and applied practice, there is consensus about its core tenets. HFE practice is fundamentally about designing sociotechnical systems and should always:

(1) take a systems approach
(2) aim to design interactions
(3) focus on two closely related outcomes, that is, system performance and human well-being.

With these historical roots and disciplinary foundations in mind, the next section explores how HFE has evolved within, and has been applied to, the healthcare domain.

2.2 Healthcare Human Factors and Ergonomics

As discussed in the previous section, HFE is fundamentally concerned with the design of interactions in sociotechnical systems to enhance system performance and human well-being. Healthcare presents a compelling but complex setting for the application of HFE approaches.

2.2.1 Physical Ergonomics

One of the early areas where HFE was applied in healthcare was physical ergonomics during the 1990s, particularly in the design of buildings, equipment, and systems to prevent musculoskeletal disorders among healthcare workers.[12] Work in operating theatres, midwifery, physiotherapy, radiography, and ambulance services is often repetitive, requires similar movements and postures for extended periods of time, and frequently involves lifting heavy loads. In nursing and allied health professions, manual patient handling represents a major musculoskeletal risk, and the application of physical ergonomics has been shown to be an effective approach for assessing and mitigating such risks.[13]

Posture analysis studies using HFE techniques, such as Rapid Upper Limb Assessment (RULA) and Rapid Entire Body Assessment (REBA), have shown how patient-handling tasks are associated with high rates of harmful postures, particularly when staff are unable to modify their environment or the patient's position.[14] Reviews of the literature highlighted the limited value of traditional manual handling education alone, which has little long-term impact on injury rates.[15,16] Instead, multifactorial interventions that combine equipment provision, risk assessment, redesign of the work environment, and changes to work organisation – alongside training – are most likely to succeed.[12]

2.2.2 Usability of Medical Devices and Health Information Technology

In parallel, the 1990s and 2000s saw increasing attention to HFE in the design and use of medical devices and health information technology (IT), particularly around usability and patient safety. Studies demonstrated that technologies, such as computerised physician order entry systems, barcoded medication administration systems, and electronic health records, could introduce unanticipated consequences and new types of errors.[17,18] These systems have also been associated with increased staff fatigue and cognitive burden.[19]

The medical device industry is subject to extensive regulation, and the application of usability engineering principles is supported by dedicated standards. IEC 62366 (Medical Devices – Application of Usability Engineering to Medical Devices), first published in 2007 and revised in 2015, sets out processes for applying usability engineering to medical devices. More generally, ISO 92411–11 (Ergonomics of Human–System Interaction) defines usability as the 'extent to which a system, product or service can be used by specified users to achieve specified goals with effectiveness, efficiency and satisfaction in a specified context of use'. Usability, therefore, is clearly set out as an attribute of a particular situation, rather than as a characteristic of the product (e.g. a medical device) by itself – again, highlighting the HFE principle of focusing on interactions.

While usability remains central in the design of medical devices and health IT, modern applications of HFE typically extend beyond this to consider the diversity of deployment contexts and the dynamic nature of healthcare. The context of use often differs from what was assumed during design (work-as-imagined), and attention must be paid to how people interact with the technology on a day-to-day basis (work-as-done): for example, through enabling staff to report and discuss necessary workarounds.[20,21]

2.2.3 Teamwork and Non-Technical Skills Training

HFE in healthcare is often equated with teamwork and non-technical skills training to address communication failures, decision-making under pressure, and coordination in high-stakes environments. This strand of HFE was heavily influenced by aviation, particularly Crew Resource Management (CRM), which was adapted for healthcare, especially in anaesthesia and critical care.[22] CRM-style training approaches, such as Team Strategies and Tools to Enhance Performance and Patient Safety (TeamSTEPPS),[23] have been shown to improve teamwork behaviours and key processes.

However, training in isolation is reductionist and limiting, considering that in aviation and other industries, teamwork training is only one aspect of wider human factors integration.[24] A systems-oriented HFE perspective views teamwork as an emergent outcome of interactions of the elements of a work system, rather than as a set of skills residing within individuals.[1] For example, effective layout of workspaces can enable communication through shared spaces or reduce the need for unnecessary communication (e.g. having a clear line of sight to shared information), thereby reducing interruptions.

2.2.4 Accident Models and Contributory Factors Frameworks

The mainstream patient safety movement gained momentum around the turn of the millennium, catalysed by the influential Institute of Medicine report 'To err is human'.[26] The report helped shift the dominant view of safety from one focused on human error and individual blame to one that emphasised system failures and contributory factors. Psychologist James Reason's work was central to this transformation.

Reason's Swiss cheese model offered a compelling graphical explanation of how accidents arise from multiple interacting failures, both at the sharp end (unsafe acts), as well as at the so-called blunt end (latent conditions).[11] Reason argued that an effective safety management strategy should improve the conditions under which people work, rather than trying to 'fix' the human condition, that is, get people to make fewer errors.[27]

The hierarchy of controls approach provides a simple classification of safety barriers and risk controls based on their perceived strength, with design-based controls considered stronger than behaviour-based controls. Hazards should be eliminated or substituted where possible, followed by engineering controls, and then consideration of policies, work instructions, and personal protective equipment. Direct transfer of a hierarchy of risk controls from safety-critical industries to healthcare is, however, not necessarily appropriate in every context.[28]

Reason's ideas inspired the development of structured methods for understanding contributory factors in healthcare, such as the London Protocol (a method of investigating clinical incidents in healthcare).[29] It also encouraged the widespread adoption of incident-reporting systems, such as the National Reporting and Learning System (NRLS) and the Learning from Patient Safety Events Service (LfPSE) in the National Health Service (NHS).[30]

2.2.5 Safety Culture

Reason's approach to safety management is underpinned by the concept of safety culture, which includes the interrelated notions of reporting culture, just culture, flexible culture, and learning culture.[11] Healthcare organisations and regulators have adopted these ideas to foster incident-reporting, learning from failures and leadership commitment to safety. This is often supported by quantitative or semi-quantitative safety culture assessment tools, such as the Safety Attitudes Questionnaire (SAQ) or the Manchester Patient Safety Assessment Framework (MaPSaF).[31,32]

There are, however, important limitations to treating safety culture as a single organisational attribute that can be measured or changed through top-down programmes.[33] Healthcare organisations typically contain multiple professional and departmental subcultures, and culture is expressed in everyday work practices and relationships, as much as in formal statements of values. As a result, culture-change initiatives often have slow and uneven effects, and the evidence linking them directly to improvements in patient safety remains limited.[33]

Alongside these debates, the concept of restorative practice – for example, as part of restorative just culture – has received increased attention.[34,35] Harm from a patient safety incident can be aggravated by an organisation's inappropriate or exclusionary response. Restorative practice focuses on the healing and repair of relationships following patient safety incidents.

2.2.6 Complex Systems Frameworks

As the Swiss cheese model began to shape thinking about patient safety in healthcare, this period also saw more explicit interdisciplinary efforts to design safer healthcare systems, shaped by an emerging understanding of complexity, interdependence, and the importance of HFE, as well as other disciplines such as design.[36]

The growing recognition of the intricate and dynamic nature of healthcare systems has led to the adoption of systems approaches for improving the quality and safety of care. One such systems approach is the Systems Engineering Initiative for Patient Safety (SEIPS) model, which focuses on interactions between people, tasks, tools, and technologies, and the physical, organisational, and wider socioeconomic and regulatory environments.[37,38]

Another example is resilient healthcare,[39] which builds on principles of resilience engineering.[40] Resilience engineering highlights that risks can arise not only from potential failures of individual system elements but also from the structure and interconnectedness of the systems themselves. Resilience has been defined as the ability to succeed under varying conditions, focussing on how people and organisations adapt to complexity and uncertainty in real-world settings.[41] The concept of resilience includes four core abilities, or resilience potentials:[42,43]

(1) monitoring
(2) responding

(3) anticipating
(4) learning.

In healthcare, this has been interpreted as the ability to adapt to challenges and changes across different levels of a system in order to maintain high-quality care.[44]

This perspective shifts attention from traditional safety strategies focused on preventing failure (e.g. barriers and defences) to a more proactive orientation centred on enabling adaptive capacity. The Safety-II perspective was introduced to clarify this distinction – contrasting with the conventional Safety-I approach, which focuses on what goes wrong – with a view that also considers why things go right under varying conditions.[45] While resilient healthcare and Safety-II approaches have been met with enthusiasm by many working in patient safety, their practical application remains a work in progress.[46,47]

2.2.7 NHS Policy Developments

In the NHS in England, patient safety policy has increasingly embraced systems thinking and HFE principles to better focus on whole-system design, collaborative learning, and compassionate support for patients, carers, and staff.[48] The NHS Patient Safety Strategy comprises several interlinked components, including the national Patient Safety Syllabus and the Patient Safety Incident Response Framework (PSIRF).[35,49]

Introduced in 2022 to replace the Serious Incident Framework, PSIRF was developed in response to longstanding concerns about the limitations of traditional root cause analysis in healthcare safety investigations.[50,51] In contrast, PSIRF encourages the use of systems-based approaches, such as SEIPS, to guide patient safety incident response. It also places emphasis on compassionate engagement with those affected by patient safety incidents and on reducing compounded harm from the learning response itself.

2.2.8 Healthcare AI

As health systems respond to demographic changes and economic pressures, one of the most significant recent developments is the rapid integration of artificial intelligence (AI).[52] This creates both challenges and opportunities for HFE, particularly under the umbrella of human-centred (healthcare) AI.[53,54]

The dominant design paradigm has often been AI-centric, aiming to develop AI models that outperform humans in tasks traditionally performed by people.[55] Examples range from image-analysis algorithms to systems detecting cardiac arrest from emergency calls or performing well on medical examinations.[56–59]

These AI systems are typically evaluated based on retrospective algorithmic accuracy, with currently far fewer studies examining how AI performs once embedded in the realities of clinical practice.[60]

This is problematic because the performance, usability, and safety of AI technologies can only reliably be assessed in real-world settings, where interactions between people, tasks, technology, and environments shape outcomes.[61] For example, autonomous devices such as AI-supported infusion pumps may free clinicians for direct patient care, but they may also shift roles towards remote monitoring and supervision, potentially distancing staff from patients.[62]

In recognition of these challenges, CIEHF (Chartered Institute of Ergonomics and Human Factors) published a white paper on 'Human Factors and Ergonomics in Healthcare AI', which sets out a systems-based HFE vision for healthcare AI.[63] It addresses a range of critical issues, including situation awareness, impact on workload, reliance on AI technology, explanation and trust, human–AI teaming, stakeholder training, the impact on relationships between people, and the ethical dimensions of AI integration.[64] As AI becomes increasingly embedded in healthcare, sustained HFE involvement will be essential to ensure these technologies are usable, ethical, and aligned with the realities of clinical work.

2.2.9 Summary

In summary, the breadth of models and methods means there is no single HFE approach – rather the discipline represents a diverse and evolving set of practices informed by insights from multiple fields. What distinguishes HFE, as reflected in the IEA definition, is the explicit consideration of context, the focus on understanding and designing interactions, and the aim of improving system performance and human well-being. Emerging challenges, such as the growing integration of AI into sociotechnical systems, will continue to test and expand the boundaries of HFE, particularly in relation to ethics, trust, and value alignment. These core principles, however, remain a vital foundation.

3 Human Factors and Ergonomics in Action

HFE is a practical discipline in which professionals and practitioners apply scientific evidence and system-based methods to improve the everyday problems experienced by people. In healthcare, a 2020 publication estimated that there were fewer than five professionally qualified HFE specialists employed across NHS Trusts – approximately one per 300,000 staff.[65] Although some additional posts have since been created, overall HFE capacity in the NHS remains very small.

As noted, much of the recorded HFE work in healthcare starts around the 1990s, with rapid growth since then in both research and practice. This section describes selected examples of healthcare HFE from the 1990s to the present day. Each example gives an insight into the problem, approach, and output of the HFE work. The examples have been selected to illustrate how HFE is used to analyse and design different types of interactions in healthcare, such as between people and their physical environment, between users and medical devices, or between clinical teams and organisational systems.

3.1 HFE Approaches to the Design of Clinical Environments

Early applications of HFE in healthcare focused on physical ergonomics and the design of clinical environments. Healthcare spaces are often inherited rather than purpose-designed, and staff have limited ability to modify them in the context of their work. Poorly designed environments can create avoidable risks and hidden costs, while HFE can provide evidence to support redesign and business cases for change.[66]

3.1.1 The Problem

National design guidance for healthcare space requirements was not always aligned with the realities of clinical work. Evidence was needed to specify functional space requirements for activities in areas such as critical care and neonatal intensive care.[67]

3.1.2 The Approach

Over more than two decades, Hignett and colleagues developed and applied a five-step protocol using a multi-method HFE approach to inform national guidance on functional space.[68] 'Functional space' refers to the size of area required for completion of functional activities relative to the people, tasks, and equipment required.

The five-step protocol provides a useful illustration of typical HFE professional practice:

Step 1 – define an example for testing taken from either existing guidelines or real-life examples with differing dimensions and layout. This will provide a 'real-life' layout mock-up for testing.

Step 2 – use observations and create a hierarchical task analysis and link analysis to record and develop a representative scenario to test, based on the frequency or criticality of tasks.

Step 3 – conduct functional space experiments using the outputs from steps 1 and 2 to evaluate the functional requirements. Functional requirements include the number of staff, equipment required and space occupied.

Step 4 – consider additional requirements, for example, storage, family rooms, and national recommendations.

Step 5 – use steps 1–4 to test the special dimensions to support changes to work practices or the introduction of equipment or technology.

Two fundamental HFE methods are mentioned as part of this approach: hierarchical task analysis and link analysis (see Sujan et al., 2025[1] for further details on both).

(1) Hierarchical task analysis – one of the most common HFE methods used to break down the activities required to achieve a high-level system or process goal. It has been found to be useful to study clinical tasks.[69]

(2) Link analysis – a technique for analysing movements between individuals and system elements, based on observable or measurable data to represent the nature and frequency of the links. This may include movement or interactions of people with people, people in their environment with equipment, or with the interface of a device.

The protocol was applied to the design of functional spaces in critical care and neonatal intensive care units (CICU/NICU), where space constraints and increasing technological demands can compromise care delivery. Existing layouts from real units were recreated in full-scale mock-ups, enabling clinicians to engage with familiar tasks in controlled but realistic conditions. The resulting data from the application of the five-step protocol supported the refinement of space specifications, ensuring alignment between actual workflow demands and the dimensions recommended in national design guidance.

3.1.3 Output

The findings informed national guidance and contributed to the redesign of local critical care and neonatal facilities. Over the past 15 years, this approach has been adapted to address a variety of healthcare design challenges. The growing body of evidence around physical HFE practice has deepened understanding of how to align healthcare environments with the needs and interactions of those delivering and receiving care.[70,71]

For example, Kwok and Lam applied a similar systems-based methodology to reduce patient falls.[72] Likewise, a study focused on anaesthetist workspace design used HFE methods in the review of critical tasks and movements of staff, equipment location, interactions with the patient and other team members, and the physical space available.[73]

These examples highlight how the use of HFE has matured into a well-established practice in healthcare environment design, demonstrating sustained relevance and value across diverse clinical settings.

3.2 HFE Approaches to Designing and Procuring Medical Devices and Technology

The development and implementation of digital solutions and medical devices are now central to healthcare and patient safety.[74] HFE methods have been used to support both device development and procurement by focusing on usability, cognitive demands, and the wider work system.

3.2.1 The Problem

In neonatal resuscitation, timely and accurate heart rate information is critical, yet existing monitoring methods (such as auscultation with a stethoscope) can be slow, inaccurate, and disruptive.[75,76] There was a need for more reliable, usable continuous heart rate monitoring during time-critical interventions.

3.2.2 The Approach

Pickup and colleagues used HFE methods to inform the interface design of a new device for continuous heart rate monitoring during neonatal resuscitation.[77] A user-centred design process combined applied cognitive task analysis (ACTA) with expert consultation and simulation.[78] In contrast to hierarchical task analysis, ACTA focuses on cognitive demands rather than on observable actions.

ACTA has four key stages:

(1) Task diagramming – interviews with clinicians and a review of training materials supported the development of a task diagram representing key tasks and critical or difficult cognitive work associated with newborn resuscitation.
(2) Knowledge elicitation – interviews with neonatal experts probed expert knowledge of newborn resuscitation to consider decision-making cues, potential sources of errors, and strategies that distinguish expert from novice performance (see Box 1).
(3) Simulation workshop – stakeholders, including neonatal nurses and doctors, participated in simulated scenarios to explore task cognitive requirements, information needs, and contextual factors affecting performance.

Box 1: Cognitive demands and requirements summary

Why is it difficult?

(1) Interpretation of heart rate and chest movement relative to normal parameters.
(2) Judgement of the accuracy and reliability of the heart rate display.
(3) Reliance on previous experience and recognition of 'normal' heart rate and chest movement to inform decisions and actions.
(4) Multiple tasks in a short timeframe: visual check of heart rate, chest movement, tone, and skin colour. Continual re-evaluation every 30 seconds.
(5) Requires expertise to ensure decision-making within a short time-frame and potentially stressful environment.

Common errors

(1) Accuracy in interpretation of heart rate.
(2) Fail to recall normal heart rate and chest movement.
(3) Estimation/recall of time elapsed between key events.
(4) Failure to recognise when to act (e.g. call for help and intubation).
(5) Avoidance behaviour: fear to act/'failure to rescue'.
(6) Overreliance on technology (lacking reliability) and colleagues' earlier assessment.
(7) Quiet breathing missed (e.g. preterm babies).
(8) Lighting can distort baby colour.

Cues

(1) Absent heart rate, heart rate < 60 beats/minute.
(2) Heart rate > 100 beats/minute.
(3) Floppy.
(4) White colouring.
(5) No breathing/gasping.
(6) Stressful environment.
(7) Absence of baby crying.

Strategies

(1) Consider how to obtain support with minimal alarm to the parent.
(2) Continually question the interpretation/reliability of information.
(3) Continual reassessment at 30 seconds and after 1, 5, and 10 minutes.
(4) Closer inspection (e.g. ear to mouth), observe rib cage and abdomen, listen for absence of sound or gasping.

(4) Cognitive demands and requirements summary – insights were consolidated into a table of cognitive demands, summarising key user needs for interface design. An example of the details contained within the cognitive demand table is in Box 1.

Given that live observation of newborn resuscitation was not feasible, the study drew on training materials, simulation footage, and expert validation throughout.

3.2.3 Output

The study identified a range of user requirements shaped by the interactions between the tasks, roles, equipment, and the care environment. These included:

(1) Portability and vibration resistance of the system to support continued monitoring as the baby is moved.
(2) Flexibility of the positioning of the device and interface to allow movement and rotation to improve the line of sight for clinicians involved.
(3) Illumination of the screen to be able to accommodate room lighting, which may be dimmed or bright depending on the situation.
(4) Alarm type, frequency, and pitch are to be considered to avoid unintended consequences for both families and clinicians.
(5) Compatibility with other equipment required during newborn resuscitation.

These insights also shifted the overall device design from an initially planned multifunctional interface towards a simpler display, better suited to high-stress, time-critical use. The work illustrates how HFE methods can challenge design assumptions and support usability and situation awareness in medical device development.

Carman and colleagues also illustrate how similar HFE approaches can support procurement and usability testing for technologies such as hospital beds and mattresses.[79] Although these devices are not highly complex, the diversity of patient needs creates complexity in selection and implementation.

The need for stronger HFE involvement in digital health is also growing. In the UK, digital clinical safety standards DCB0129 and DCB0160 set out requirements for risk management in health IT systems. While they do not explicitly mention HFE, they imply many of its principles, such as usability, safety, and error mitigation. However, without sufficient HFE, these standards may be applied without fully addressing cognitive demands, or interface design or system-level interactions.[80]

3.3 HFE Approaches to Designing System Changes for Safety Improvement

Improving patient safety often requires interventions that go beyond isolated fixes to address the underlying complexity of healthcare systems.[81] HFE can complement and strengthen existing quality improvement and transformation efforts by applying systems thinking and participatory design methods.[82] These approaches are particularly valuable because many safety-related risks are shaped by workflows, technology, organisational practices, the physical environment, and external influences, including targets, workforce strategies, and funding decisions.[83]

3.3.1 The Problem

Misidentification of patients is a longstanding problem for healthcare providers.[84] In radiology, this can lead to the wrong patient receiving an examination, unintended radiation exposure, and delays. In 2023–2024, there were 819 notifications of accidental or unintended exposure to radiation reported to the Care Quality Commission (CQC), with patient misidentification a recurring contributory factor.[85]

3.3.2 The Approach

Woodward and colleagues observed that annual CQC reports typically framed frontline staff as the sole cause.[86] This view fails to reflect the systems thinking principles that underpin HFE. In response, they conducted a systems-focused study at a large teaching hospital in England to examine patient misidentification aligned to HFE thinking.

Using the SEIPS framework as a guiding structure,[87] the study applied a range of HFE methods to examine everyday radiography work and the trade-offs staff make to balance efficiency of the service with an acceptable level of safety. Interactions were examined at three levels using a participatory approach:

(1) Micro level – structured field observations in the control room were used to study interactions between the operator, communication tasks, and the work environment.
(2) Unit level – task analysis and hazard analysis (Failure Mode and Effects Analysis)[88] were carried out on the patient identification procedure to understand the discrete tasks and equipment interactions that support the operator to correctly identify the patient.
(3) Organisational level – scenario-based system analysis workshops – underpinned by SEIPS – explored trade-offs, interactions of the team, tasks, and reporting practices.

This layered, participatory approach enabled a richer understanding of how interactions across the system influenced behaviour at the frontline and supported the design of context-sensitive safety improvement interventions.

3.3.3 Output

The study led to a set of complementary interventions:

(1) At the *micro level*, measures to reduce distractions and interruptions, for example, updating the hospital phone directory to divert calls away from the control room.
(2) At the *unit level*, a single standard operating procedure and visualisation for patient identification based on user-centred design principles.
(3) At the *organisational level*, HFE education was delivered across the radiology teams based on the SEIPS framework to support systems thinking, encourage near-miss reporting and support discussions around the challenge of patient identification.

The study found a statistically significant increase in near-miss reporting and a significant improvement in the reduction of interruptions within the control room over a two-year period.

In other studies, SEIPS was used to improve the design of cardiac diagnostic services in community settings,[89] and to inform analysis of readmission of surgical patients at a paediatric hospital.[90]

3.4 HFE Approaches to Learning from Incidents

Health systems have been encouraged to become learning organisations. Following the inquiry into the failings at Mid Staffordshire NHS Foundation Trust, the Berwick report challenged the NHS to become an organisation dedicated to learning and continuous improvement.[91] Across safety-critical industries, learning from incidents is a key component of safety management systems. Modern approaches incorporate HFE and systems thinking, going beyond narrow consideration of 'human error' to consider the breadth of interactions across the work system.[92]

3.4.1 The Problem

The history of oversimplifying 'root causes' of healthcare incidents has failed to reflect system theories that recognise the complexity of healthcare systems and how safety is considered an emergent property of the interactions between all elements of the system.[93] A systems approach to learning from incidents can support a just culture and more meaningful learning, replacing the traditional approach that focused on proximal factors, often resulting in interventions aimed at the individual and blaming staff for errors.[26,42]

3.4.2 The Approach

An influential system model for understanding dynamic risk management is Rasmussen's framework, which describes how decisions and pressures at multiple system levels interact to shape safety or produce accidents (see Figure 1).[94] The model reminds us that safety is a multidisciplinary endeavour, because understanding decisions at different levels of a system falls within the remit of diverse disciplines, including engineering, HFE, organisation science, law, economics and political science, and sociology. Rasmussen suggests that rather than viewing safety management as a top-down approach flowing from safety regulations and rules through to work at the sharp end, it should be reframed as a dynamic control problem, where the interaction of different pressures and constraints can gradually move a system towards and across the threshold of safe performance.

AcciMap is the method for the analysis of incidents and accidents developed from this model.[95] Capturing the wider interactions across the system to understand adverse outcomes, it is increasingly used for healthcare investigations.[96] AcciMap visualises contributory factors located at different system levels and the links between them, helping to shift attention from the 'sharp end' to the broader system context.

This method was used to investigate cross-organisational factors contributing to violence and aggression in hospital settings,[97] aiming to avoid 'safety clutter': i.e. practices that do not actually contribute to improving safety,[98] or blaming individuals for incidents.

The investigation consisted of three stages:

Stage 1. ActorMap development – Identifying 98 stakeholders across different levels of the system who influence the management of violence and aggression.

Stage 2. AcciMap construction – Mapping contributory factors across the system levels.

Stage 3. PreventiMap design – PreventiMap is based on the same visualisation of an AcciMap.[99] The intention is to visualise and co-design a set of system-level interventions linked across levels.

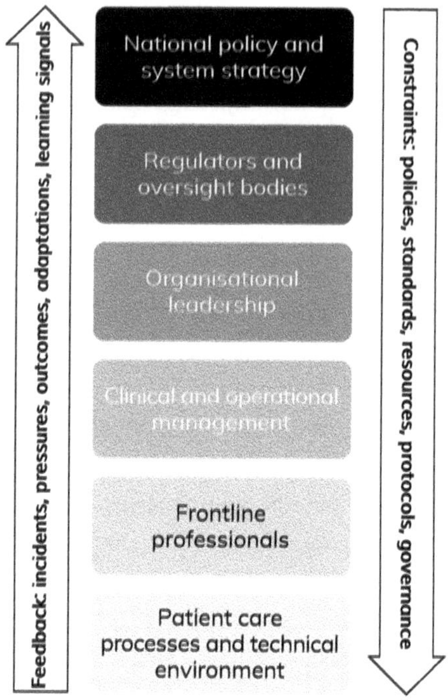

Figure 1 A healthcare-specific interpretation of Rasmussen's multi-level system for safety management. National policy decisions, regulatory requirements, and organisational priorities shape the conditions of clinical work, while signals from frontline practice and patient care processes feedback to influence decision-making at higher levels. Safety emerges from the dynamic interaction of these layers.

3.4.3 Output

The investigation showed that many stakeholders carry responsibility for managing violence and aggression, but few hold decision-making power. It highlighted interdependencies between legislation, budgeting, workforce, local management, frontline practice, and patient- and environment-related factors, and concluded that improvement would require coordinated interventions across multiple levels.

The study concluded that improvement in the management of violence and aggression would require multiple interventions that are focused across the levels of the system. The themes highlighted in the final workshop identified several areas influential to safety, including risk management, staffing, incident response, incident-reporting and learning systems, consultation and coordination across system levels, and the design of hospital environments.

This work has contributed to the New South Wales government's guidance on the management of violence and aggression, providing a practical toolkit from the findings to support safety improvement initiatives in this area.[100]

The AcciMap method is included in the NHS England Patient Safety Syllabus, and it is part of the repertoire of methods used by the Health Services Safety Investigations Body (HSSIB). It provides a way of learning from patient safety incidents by revealing interactions across different levels of complex health systems.

3.5 HFE Approaches for Proactive Safety Investigations

The English HSSIB was established in 2017 (as the Healthcare Safety Investigation Branch), with corresponding legislation introduced in 2022. HSSIB has contributed to the embedding of HFE approaches and methods in the NHS through education.

3.5.1 The Problem

Healthcare predominantly focuses on learning from past incidents. In other safety-critical industries, this practice is supported by proactive safety investigations. These can provide a dynamic approach to organisational learning on inherent hazards and risks that can be found through observing everyday work and performance.[101]

3.5.2 The Approach

During the COVID-19 pandemic, a rapid proactive safety investigation was completed and shared with the English healthcare system between the first and second waves of the pandemic in England. This was the first proactive safety investigation by HSSIB, which was intended to support real-time response to the emerging risks.

The investigation applied the SEIPS framework to support the collection of information and frame the analysis to understand systemic factors interacting and presenting as influential to the nosocomial (healthcare-associated) transmission of the virus in hospitals. The investigation combined:

(1) interviews with staff and patients
(2) observations in clinical settings
(3) a review of national and organisational guidance and documentation.

The analysis highlighted the limitations in existing practices of risk management and the impact of complex arrangements and the lack of clarity of processes to develop national guidance. The impact of the higher-level system on local practices and capability was impeded by the lack of communication on a '... single national message ...'.[102] The application of this HFE-informed proactive safety investigation provided timely learning on the system interactions influential to safety across healthcare organisations.

3.5.3 Output

The investigation produced a set of prompts for organisations to review local approaches to risk management, including governance structures, communication pathways, and support for staff. It exemplified how HFE-informed proactive investigations can provide an 'up and out' view of system interactions, complementing traditional incident investigation.

HFE methods, such as SEIPS, are now increasingly embedded in English healthcare safety work through HSSIB education and PSIRF guidance. This supports a shift away from linear and blame-oriented investigations that developed in the use of a root cause analysis approach towards system-based approaches.[81] However, it should be noted that in 2026 HSSIB terminated its education function to focus on undertaking investigations rather than contributing to building capacity.

4 Critical Reflection on Human Factors and Ergonomics as an Approach to Healthcare Improvement

While HFE offers a powerful set of concepts and methods to support safer, more effective, and more human-centred healthcare, its uptake and application have not been without challenges. As with any discipline that crosses boundaries and engages with complex systems, HFE is vulnerable to misinterpretation, oversimplification, and underutilisation. This section reflects on some of the key conceptual, practical, and structural barriers that have limited the impact of HFE in healthcare improvement efforts. It also considers deeper questions about the nature of evidence, value, and meaning in applying HFE to real-world healthcare systems. The aim is not to diminish the contribution of HFE, but to offer a constructive critique that helps clarify what is needed for its fuller, more effective integration.

4.1 Conceptual and Disciplinary Ambiguities

In the introduction, we approached HFE via the IEA definition, which provides a robust starting point. While there is widespread agreement on core tenets –

such as systems thinking, design orientation, and the dual aim of enhancing system performance and human well-being – there is less clarity when it comes to how HFE is understood and operationalised in practice.[4] This lack of shared understanding becomes particularly visible in interdisciplinary settings like healthcare, where different stakeholders encounter HFE from different sources, ranging from pilots delivering aviation-style teamwork training, research literature based on other industries, and the occasional HFE-practitioner-led design project.

The field of HFE is inherently multidisciplinary. Its intellectual roots come from psychology, anatomy, and physiology, though it also includes contributions from disciplines such as engineering, industrial design, and organisation science. As a result, it has been described variously as a scientific discipline, a design practice, a methodological toolkit, or a professional identity.[103,104] This plurality has allowed HFE to adapt across domains – for example, the military, office business settings, safety-critical industries, consumer technology, and healthcare – but it was also accompanied by confusion about the nature of the discipline. In the absence of a clear boundary or universally recognised scope, HFE is often shaped by the institutional context in which it is used.[105] In healthcare, for example, HFE may be presented as a behavioural safety intervention, as a way to support technology usability, or as an approach to understanding work-as-done. While each of these interpretations has merit, they represent only partial expressions of what HFE as a whole encompasses.[83]

A related issue is the blurring of boundaries between HFE and adjacent domains such as quality improvement, safety science, systems engineering, implementation science, and human-centred design. These overlaps can be productive, fostering collaboration and innovation.[82] However, they also carry the risk of conceptual dilution. HFE may be invoked rhetorically to signal user focus or systemic insight, even when projects lack the methodological rigour, participatory design processes, or contextual sensitivity that characterise HFE practice. In some cases, human factors become a label that is retrofitted to justify a predetermined solution, rather than a guiding influence on problem definition and intervention design.[106]

This conceptual ambiguity has practical consequences. It can lead to unrealistic expectations, either overestimating what HFE can achieve or dismissing it as too vague or 'soft'. It complicates education and training in HFE of the healthcare workforce, as there is no clearly defined pathway into HFE practice in healthcare, and there are few structures to support interdisciplinary understanding, even though there are positive developments with, for example, the national Patient Safety Syllabus and PSIRF in the NHS in England and the CIEHF Healthcare Human Factors Learning Pathway. Conceptual ambiguity also undermines efforts to integrate HFE into organisational strategy, policy, and procurement. In contrast to industries in which HFE is embedded in safety regulation and design processes from the outset, healthcare systems often struggle to make sustained use of HFE expertise.

Clarifying the distinctive principles of HFE – such as the focus on systems, design of interactions, and the commitment to enhancing both system performance and human well-being – remains a key challenge for the field. Without this clarity, the promise of HFE as a driver of improvement in healthcare will continue to be constrained by conceptual ambiguity and fragmentation.

4.2 Misapplication and Practical Challenges

Human Factors and Ergonomics is often applied narrowly and superficially because the infrastructure, literacy, and positioning for deeper application are lacking. As described earlier, HFE is frequently reduced to 'the human factors approach', with a focus on communication and teamwork training. Worse still, HFE is also sometimes misrepresented as 'the human factor', that is, as the cause of adverse events, where subsequent 'improvement' interventions are targeted at the level of the individual through behavioural safety programmes. The risk is that this reductionist framing neglects the inherent systems perspective and design focus of HFE, misleading people into assuming that training and behavioural safety are sufficient to address performance and well-being in complex systems.[4,83]

Such reductionist applications of HFE are often symptoms of more structural barriers and practical challenges. One of these is the lack of available HFE expertise. In the UK and the US, for example, there are few chartered ergonomists (or similarly qualified individuals) working in the health sector, and most healthcare organisations have no in-house HFE expertise at all.[107] While clinical enthusiasts may have an awareness of HFE, they might lack sufficient experience in the broader discipline and the requirements for its successful application in practice. Frequently, HFE considerations are then brought in at a late stage, for example, after technology procurement decisions have been made and problems in use have been reported.

The lack of systematic mechanisms for HFE integration further compounds this problem. In industries such as aviation, railways, and nuclear energy, HFE is embedded in regulation, procurement, and design processes. The regulatory support and formal guidance for HFE integration have supported the development and deployment of HFE expertise across these industries. Such HFE integration mechanisms are largely absent in healthcare.

Without clarity in processes and a strategy to embed HFE within existing healthcare processes, the potential for HFE application might not be realised, limiting its contribution to improving patient safety, staff well-being, and overall system performance. The role of HFE must be reimagined: it should be seen not as a reactive and narrow fix, but as a proactive and foundational perspective embedded early and consistently in the design, evaluation, and improvement of healthcare systems. Such HFE integration would benefit from compelling narratives about the contribution of HFE to the quality and safety of healthcare and the well-being of staff. This raises questions about what counts as credible evidence for HFE in healthcare, and how its value can be articulated within the decision-making logics of healthcare organisations as businesses.

4.3 The Nature of Evidence

One of the major challenges facing HFE in healthcare is the relative lack of rigorous evaluation studies. Despite wide recognition of its conceptual value and a growing number of applications in healthcare, HFE still lacks a convincing and coherent evidence base that demonstrates the effectiveness of its application in practice.[115] While this lack of evidence has not prevented the adoption of HFE in safety-critical industries, it is a significant limiting factor in healthcare, where there is a greater focus on underpinning interventions with evidence.

Consider, for example, the concept of safety cases, which is a regulatory approach for assuring and demonstrating that a system (such as a nuclear power plant) is acceptably safe to operate under specific conditions. Despite decades of academic reflection on the structure, content, and format of safety cases, there is a near-total absence of evaluation in healthcare – calling into question their value.[108,109] Similarly, the field of Safety-II and the associated Functional Resonance Analysis Method (FRAM) have become increasingly popular across industries, including healthcare.[110] However, corresponding studies often do not attempt, or struggle, to demonstrate that systems and well-being have been improved as a result of interventions rooted in this thinking.[46] The challenge for HFE researchers and practitioners is to articulate explicitly the theories or logic models for proposed interventions so that claims about how to improve system performance and human well-being – and under what circumstances – can be critically appraised.

In this respect, healthcare may offer a more fertile ground than many of the other safety-critical industries, even if the evidence base for healthcare quality improvement struggles with similar challenges.[111] Over the past two decades, considerable progress has been made in the development of frameworks for the evaluation of complex interventions, most notably the updated guidance issued by the Medical Research Council and the National Institute for Health and Care Excellence (NICE).[112] This framework recognises that interventions often have multiple interacting components, that context shapes outcomes, and that causal mechanisms need to be made explicit and testable.

Whether the Medical Research Council/NICE framework provides an exact fit for the evaluation of HFE interventions remains to be investigated. HFE practice is often not based on delivering a discrete intervention, but on facilitating the design of interactions in sociotechnical systems. This work is frequently embedded in ongoing change processes, it involves negotiation and adaptation, and there might not be clearly delineated start and end points. Moreover, outcomes may be emergent, non-linear and hard to quantify, such as increased resilience and improved ability to respond to changing contexts. While the general principles for evaluating complex interventions remain valuable and go beyond current practice in HFE (and safety science), complementary approaches may offer additional insight into how complex changes unfold in practice. These include realist evaluation, ethnographic or mixed-method process evaluations, and theory-driven approaches such as normalisation process theory, which seeks to explain how complex interventions become embedded.[113–115]

A further set of challenges concerns the quality and accumulation of evidence. As Dixon-Woods notes, healthcare improvement is often carried out as small, local projects with limited methodological rigour, weak theorisation, and inadequate reporting.[116] As a result, it is often difficult to determine whether an intervention worked, why it worked, or whether it could work elsewhere. Too often, improvement studies fail to articulate clear mechanisms of change, use inconsistent or poorly constructed measures, or operate in ways that prevent learning from being accumulated across settings. This fragmentation means that promising approaches remain confined to local pockets of practice, while similar problems are repeatedly rediscovered or addressed anew. Following this argument, strengthening the evidence base for HFE therefore requires not only evaluating whether interventions are effective, but also improving the design, reporting, and cumulative learning of HFE work, thereby treating HFE interventions as objects of study, making their underlying logic explicit, and enabling findings to be shared, compared and refined across contexts.

The development of a more robust and credible evidence base for HFE in healthcare requires greater use of suitable evaluation approaches that reflect the realities of HFE practice. HFE researchers and practitioners should become more explicit in describing not only the motivation behind HFE interventions but also in articulating assumptions about how interventions would work, for whom, and under what conditions. Building this kind of evidence base requires a change in mindset within HFE as a discipline.

4.4 Making the Business Case for HFE

HFE aims to improve system performance and human well-being, but these benefits are rarely expressed in the language of cost, return on investment, or strategic value creation that drives health system policy and decision-making. In short, there is a lack of a compelling business case for HFE.

The nature of HFE work, as described in the previous sections, contributes to this difficulty. Many of the outcomes of the application of HFE theories, concepts, and methods are systemic, longer-term, and emergent. Examples include improved cognitive workload profiles, better coordination, and enhanced capacity to adapt to change. These are real and important contributions, but they do not always map easily onto established economic or managerial metrics. Return on investment is difficult to calculate in non-linear sociotechnical systems, and the impact of HFE interventions is rarely isolated or direct.[107] It remains challenging to translate the value of HFE into the logic of healthcare funding and health system management. This continues to create a significant obstacle to the acceptance and adoption of HFE in healthcare improvement practice.

The challenges with providing a compelling business case for HFE are not unique to healthcare. In air traffic management, the European network management agency Eurocontrol issued guidance for the business case for HFE.[117] The guidance argues that early integration of HFE in the design of air traffic management services can reduce costs by providing input at the early stages of product and service development, which can help reduce the need for later retrofitting fixes and costly redesign. Policy documents such as this can help shift the thinking from HFE as a cost towards HFE as an enabler of strategic and operational performance.

The Eurocontrol guidance emphasises that building a compelling business case for HFE requires mapping the different types of beneficiaries, as well as the different types of benefits. Producing such a map could be a helpful first step towards a healthcare business case for HFE. For example, early consideration of HFE in the design and subsequent deployment of an AI ambient digital scribe could improve clinician well-being (staff benefit), free up time for patient interaction (care quality and patient experience benefits), and reduce burnout and staff turnover (organisational benefit). However, in many such cases, HFE is considered at a late stage to troubleshoot problems, and only a small selection of, usually, quantifiable outcomes are reported. A clearer mapping of beneficiaries and benefits could support healthcare leaders and decision-makers to recognise the value of HFE investment.

This is particularly relevant in the current context of large-scale AI deployment and an increasing focus on health system learning, adaptive capacity, compassionate engagement, and staff well-being. These are areas where there is significant scope for HFE to add value. However, HFE as a discipline and a profession has not yet developed effective ways of converting conceptual alignment into strategic buy-in. There is a need for better evidence, better framing, and more willingness to engage with the economic and managerial logics that govern healthcare improvement efforts.

5 Conclusions

HFE is a scientific discipline and a professional practice concerned with designing interactions in sociotechnical systems to improve both system performance and human well-being. It takes a systems approach, is fundamentally design-oriented, and focuses on understanding and shaping the relationships between people, their tasks, the tools and technologies they use, the physical spaces, and the organisational and wider socioeconomic and regulatory environments. HFE originated from multidisciplinary efforts to solve practical problems in military operations during the Second World War. Today, HFE is a diverse and multidisciplinary field, with applications across many safety-critical industries, business and home technologies, and healthcare.

In the early 1990s, HFE in healthcare was largely confined to addressing issues related to musculoskeletal disease from manual handling and repetitive work, as well as usability issues in the use of medical devices. With the onset of the mainstream patient safety movement in the early 2000s, HFE gained greater recognition in healthcare, largely due to the adoption of aviation-style teamwork training programmes. While this represents a reductionist interpretation of HFE, it has paved the way for the more holistic application of HFE we see today. HFE is now firmly embedded in national patient safety initiatives such as the NHS Patient Safety Strategy, the PSIRF, and the NHS Patient Safety Syllabus. HFE input to the response to the COVID-19 pandemic – facilitated in the UK by the CIEHF – has raised awareness of HFE among a broader range of stakeholders across the health system.

While its role is increasingly recognised, it is still inconsistently understood and applied in practice.[24] The full potential of HFE in healthcare remains far from being clearly articulated and realised. In many areas, such as digital health and AI-enabled service delivery, there persists a technology focus, and HFE is underused – or applied too late – to shape key design and implementation decisions. There is a need for a more strategic and systematic approach to HFE integration in healthcare improvement.

Professionalisation of the HFE practitioner role in healthcare is an essential part of this journey. Continuing professional development, consistent pathways into practice, and greater awareness of HFE among senior decision-makers are all critical to ensuring that HFE expertise is understood and effectively deployed. Recent developments, such as the CIEHF Healthcare Human Factors Learning Pathway and training offered by the charity Clinical Human Factors Group (CHFG), provide encouraging examples of how this might be achieved. At the same time, HFE should be reflected in guidance, procurement frameworks, and safety standards, creating the structural conditions for meaningful HFE integration.

The HFE profession needs to embrace the challenges of HFE integration and be more responsive to the traditions and the discourse in healthcare by building a stronger evidence base and developing a more compelling business case. While the complexity of HFE work makes standard evaluation challenging, it is essential that HFE researchers and practitioners become more explicit about how interventions are expected to bring about change, for whom, and under what conditions. Alongside this, more attention must be paid to identifying the full range of HFE beneficiaries and the diverse forms of value HFE can offer: from improving usability, and reducing injuries and harm, to enhancing patient experience and staff well-being, as well as enabling organisational resilience.

Further Reading

Sujan et al.[118] – An introductory text on HFE in health and social care. The material is structured around an HFE work system model (SEIPS). The focus is applied.

Carayon et al.[87] – An article describing the Systems Engineering Initiative for Patient Safety (SEIPS) framework. There are more recent descriptions, but it is useful to look at this early formulation.

Russ et al.[4] – An article discussing and explaining common HFE misinterpretations in healthcare.

Catchpole[24] – An editorial accompanying the article by Russ et al. The editorial provides a critical reflection on the adoption of aviation-style teamwork training in healthcare.

Verhagen et al.[46] – An article providing a critical reflection on the application of Safety-II in healthcare.

Wilson[103] – An article describing the principles of systems thinking in HFE. It uses a railway example.

Wilson and Sharples[119] A comprehensive book covering many aspects of HFE in around 1,000 pages, it provides a good way to get started with a certain HFE topic – simply find the corresponding chapter in the book.

Stanton et al.[104] – A reference book that contains short descriptions of a large number of HFE methods. It is not meant to be read from cover to cover. You can pick a method and get a very quick high-level overview.

Contributors

Both authors have contributed equally. Both authors have approved the final version.

Conflicts of interest

Mark Sujan is a Trustee of the Chartered Institute of Ergonomics and Human Factors, and he is an Ambassador for the Clinical Human Factors Group.

Acknowledgements

We thank the THIS Institute editorial team and the peer reviewers for their insightful comments and recommendations to improve the Element. A list of peer reviewers is published at www.cambridge.org/IQ-peer-reviewers.

Funding

This Element was funded by THIS Institute (The Healthcare Improvement Studies Institute, www.thisinstitute.cam.ac.uk). THIS Institute is strengthening the evidence base for improving the quality and safety of healthcare. THIS Institute is supported by a grant to the University of Cambridge from the Health Foundation – an independent charity committed to bringing about better health and healthcare for people in the UK.

About the Authors

Mark Sujan is Chair in Safety Science at the University of York. He is a Fellow of the Chartered Institute of Ergonomics and Human Factors, where he also serves as a Trustee on the Governing Council and as Chair of the special interest group on Digital Health & AI.

Laura Pickup is the Head of Human Factors at a large teaching hospital in Bristol and Director of an independent consultancy. She is a Fellow of the Chartered Institute of Ergonomics and Human Factors.

References

1. What is Ergonomics (HFE)? International Ergonomics Association. https://iea.cc/about/what-is-ergonomics/ (accessed 10 January 2026).
2. Jackson SL, Read GJM, Hulme A, Salmon PM. Systems human factors and Ergonomics methods: Applications, outcomes, and future directions. *Hum Factor Ergon Man* 2025; 35(3): e70002. https://doi.org/10.1002/hfm.70002.
3. Hignett S, Pascale C, Peter B, Catchpole K. State of science: Human factors and ergonomics in healthcare. *Ergonomics* 2013; 56(10): 1491–1503. https://doi.org/10.1080/00140139.2013.822932.
4. Russ AL, Fairbanks RJ, Karsh B-T, et al. The science of human factors: Separating fact from fiction. *BMJ Qual Saf* 2013; 22(10): 802–808. https://doi.org/10.1136/bmjqs-2012-001450.
5. Wilson JR. Fundamentals of ergonomics in theory and practice. *Appl Ergon* 2000; 31(6): 557–567. https://doi.org/10.1016/s0003-6870(00)00034-x.
6. Waterson P. World War II and other historical influences on the formation of the Ergonomics Research Society. *Ergonomics* 2011; 54(12): 1111–1129. https://doi.org/10.1080/00140139.2011.622796.
7. Waterson P, Eason K. '1966 and all that': Trends and developments in UK ergonomics during the 1960s. *Ergonomics* 2009; 52(11): 1323–1341. https://doi.org/10.1080/00140130903229561.
8. Waterson P, Sell R. Recurrent themes and developments in the history of the Ergonomics Society. *Ergonomics* 2006; 49(8): 743–799. https://doi.org/10.1080/00140130600676056.
9. Hollnagel E, Woods DD. Cognitive Systems Engineering: New wine in new bottles. *Int J Man-Mach Stud* 1983; 18(6): 583–600. https://doi.org/10.1016/S0020-7373(83)80034-0.
10. Perrow C. *Normal Accidents: Living with High-Risk Technologies*. London: Basic Books; 1984.
11. Reason J. *Managing the Risks of Organizational Accidents*. Farnham: Ashgate; 1997.
12. Hignett S, Fray M, Matz M. Assessment and evaluation tools for healthcare ergonomics: Musculoskeletal disorders and patient handling. In Carayon P, ed. *Handbook of Human Factors and Ergonomics in Health Care and Patient Safety*. 2nd ed. Boca Raton: CRC Press; 2012: 235–246.
13. Alexander P, Crumpton E, Fletcher B, et al. *Evidence-based patient handling: Tasks, equipment, and interventions*. Abingdon: Routledge; 2003.

14. Hignett S. Fitting the work to the Physiotherapist. *Physiotherapy* 1995; 81(9): 549–552. https://doi.org/10.1016/S0031-9406(05)66693-X.
15. Hignett S. Work-related back pain in nurses. *J Adv Nurs* 1996; 23(6): 1238–1246. https://doi.org/10.1046/j.1365-2648.1996.13423.x.
16. Hignett S. Intervention strategies to reduce musculoskeletal injuries associated with handling patients: A systematic review. *Occup Environ Med* 2003; 60(9): e6. https://doi.org/10.1136/oem.60.9.e6.
17. Ash JS, Sittig DF, Dykstra RH, et al. Categorizing the unintended sociotechnical consequences of computerized provider order entry. *Int J Med Inform* 2007; 76 Suppl 1:S21–7. https://doi.org/10.1016/j.ijmedinf.2006.05.017.
18. Koppel R, Metlay JP, Cohen A, et al. Role of computerized physician order entry systems in facilitating medication errors. *JAMA* 2005; 293(10): 1197–203. https://doi.org/10.1001/jama.293.10.1197.
19. Hill RG, Sears LM, Melanson SW. 4000 Clicks: A productivity analysis of electronic medical records in a community hospital ED. *Am J Emerg Med* 2013; 31(11): 1591–1594. https://doi.org/10.1016/j.ajem.2013.06.028.
20. Blandford A, Furniss D, Vincent C. Patient safety and interactive medical devices: Realigning work as imagined and work as done. *Clin Risk* 2014; 20(5): 107–110. https://doi.org/10.1177/1356262214556550.
21. Debono D, Braithwaite J. Workarounds in nursing practice in acute care: A case of a health care arms race? In Wears R, Hollnagel E, Braithwaite J, eds. *The Resilience of Everyday Clinical Work*. Farnham: Ashgate; 2015.
22. Gaba DM, Howard SK, Fish KJ, Smith BE, Sowb YA. Simulation-based training in Anesthesia crisis resource management (ACRM): A decade of experience. *Simul Gaming* 2001; 32(2): 175–193. https://doi.org/10.1177/104687810103200206.
23. King HB, Battles J, Baker DP, et al. TeamSTEPPS™: team strategies and tools to enhance performance and patient safety. In Henrikson K, Battles JB, Keyes MA, Grady ML, eds. *Advances in Patient Safety: New Directions and Alternative Approaches (Vol. 3: Performance and Tools)*. Rockville, MD: Agency for Healthcare Research and Quality; 2008.
24. Catchpole K. Spreading human factors expertise in healthcare: Untangling the knots in people and systems. *BMJ Qual Saf* 2013; 22(10): 793–797. https://doi.org/10.1136/bmjqs-2013-002036.
25. What is Ergonomics? International Ergonomics Association. https://iea.cc/about/what-is-ergonomics/ (accessed 10 January 2026).
26. Kohn LT, Corrigan JM, Donaldson MS. *To Err Is Human: Building a Safer Health System*. Washington, DC: The National Academies Press; 2000.
27. Reason J. Human error: Models and management. *BMJ* 2000; 320(7237): 768–70. https://doi.org/10.1136/bmj.320.7237.768.

28. Liberati EG, Peerally MF, Dixon-Woods M. Learning from high risk industries may not be straightforward: A qualitative study of the hierarchy of risk controls approach in healthcare. *Int J Qual Health Care* 2018; 30(1): 39–43. https://doi.org/10.1093/intqhc/mzx163.
29. Vincent C, Taylor-Adams S, Stanhope N. Framework for analysing risk and safety in clinical medicine. *BMJ* 1998; 316(7138): 1154–7. https://doi.org/10.1136/bmj.316.7138.1154.
30. Department of Health. *An Organisation with a Memory*. London: The Stationery Office; 2000.
31. National Patient Safety Agency. *Manchester Patient Safety Framework*. London: National Patient Safety Agency; 2006.
32. Sexton JB, Helmreich RL, Neilands TB, et al. The Safety Attitudes Questionnaire: Psychometric properties, benchmarking data, and emerging research. *BMC Health Services Res* 2006; 6: 44. https://doi.org/10.1186/1472-6963-6-44.
33. Mannion R. *Making Culture Change Happen*. Cambridge: Cambridge University Press; 2022.
34. Dekker S, Oates A, Rafferty J. *Restorative Just Culture in Practice: Implementation and Evaluation*. London: CRC Press; 2022.
35. Lounsbury O, Sujan M. Achieving a restorative Just Culture through the patient safety incident response framework. *J Patient Saf Risk Manag* 2023; 28(4): 153–155. https://doi.org/10.1177/25160435231194397.
36. Buckle P, Clarkson PJ, Coleman R, Ward J, Anderson J. Patient safety, systems design and ergonomics. *Appl Ergon* 2006; 37(4): 491–500. https://doi.org/10.1016/j.apergo.2006.04.016.
37. Carayon P, Wooldridge A, Hoonakker P, Hundt AS, Kelly M. SEIPS 3.0: Human-centered design of the patient journey for patient safety. *Appl Ergon* 2020; 84: 103033. https://doi.org/10.1016/j.apergo.2019.103033.
38. Holden RJ, Carayon P, Gurses AP, et al. SEIPS 2.0: A human factors framework for studying and improving the work of healthcare professionals and patients. *Ergonomics* 2013; 56(11): 1669–1686. https://doi.org/10.1080/00140139.2013.838643.
39. Hollnagel E, Sujan M, Braithwaite J. Resilient Health Care – Making Steady Progress. Safety Science 2019. https://doi.org/10.1016/j.ssci.2019.07.029.
40. Hollnagel E, Woods DD, Leveson N. *Resilience Engineering: Concepts and Precepts*. Aldershot: Ashgate; 2006.
41. Woods DD, Hollnagel E. Prologue: Resilience engineering concepts. In Hollnagel E, Woods DD, Leveson N, eds. *Resilience Engineering: Concepts and Precepts*. Aldershot: Ashgate; 2006.

42. Hollnagel E. Prologue: The scope of resilience engineering. In Hollnagel E, Paries J, Woods DD, Wreathall J, eds. *Resilience Engineering in Practice: A Guidebook*. Farnham: Ashgate; 2010.
43. Hollnagel E. *Safety-II in Practice: Developing the Resilience Potentials*. Abingdon: Routledge; 2018.
44. Wiig S, Aase K, Billett S, et al. Defining the boundaries and operational concepts of resilience in the resilience in healthcare research program. *BMC Health Services Res* 2020; 20(1): 330. https://doi.org/10.1186/s12913-020-05224-3.
45. Hollnagel E. *Safety-I and Safety-II*. Farnham: Ashgate; 2014.
46. Verhagen MJ, de Vos MS, Sujan M, Hamming JF. The problem with making Safety-II work in healthcare. *BMJ Qual Saf* 2022; 31: 402–408. https://doi.org/10.1136/bmjqs-2021-014396.
47. Sujan M. Safety-II. In Cox C, Hughes H, Nicholls J, eds. *Patient Safety: Emerging Applications of Safety Science*. Bridgewater: Class Professional; 2024.
48. Lounsbury O, Sujan M, Catchpole K. From compliance to collaboration: Learning from transatlantic frameworks for healthcare safety improvement. *J Patient Saf* 2024: 20(8): e118–e120. https://doi.org/10.1097/PTS.0000000000001257.
49. Spurgeon P, Sujan M, Cross S, Flanagan H. *Building Safer Healthcare Systems*. Basel: Springer; 2019.
50. Kellogg KM, Hettinger Z, Shah M, et al. Our current approach to root cause analysis: is it contributing to our failure to improve patient safety? *BMJ Qual Saf* 2017; 26(5): 381–387. https://doi.org/10.1136/bmjqs-2016-005991.
51. Peerally MF, Carr S, Waring J, Dixon-Woods M. The problem with root cause analysis. *BMJ Qual Saf* 2017: 26(5): 417–422. https://doi.org/10.1136/bmjqs-2016-005511.
52. Topol EJ. High-performance medicine: The convergence of human and artificial intelligence. *Nat Med* 2019; 25(1): 44–56. https://doi.org/10.1038/s41591-018-0300-7.
53. Shneiderman B. Human-centered artificial intelligence: Reliable, safe & trustworthy. *Int Jf Hum–Compt Interact* 2020; 36(6): 495–504. https://doi.org/10.1080/10447318.2020.1741118.
54. Andersen TO, Nunes F, Wilcox L, Coiera E, Rogers Y. Introduction to the special issue on human-centred AI in healthcare: Challenges appearing in the wild. *ACM Trans Comput-Hum Interact* 2023; 30(2): Article 25. https://doi.org/10.1145/3589961.

55. Habli I, Sujan M, Lawton T. Moving beyond the AI sales pitch – Empowering clinicians to ask the right questions about clinical AI. *Future Healthc J* 2024; 11(3): 100–179. https://doi.org/10.1016/j.fhj.2024.100179.
56. Blomberg SN, Folke F, Ersbøll AK, et al. Machine learning as a supportive tool to recognize cardiac arrest in emergency calls. *Resuscitation* 2019; 138: 322–329. https://doi.org/10.1016/j.resuscitation.2019.01.015.
57. Li L, Qin L, Xu Z, et al. Artificial intelligence distinguishes COVID-19 from community acquired pneumonia on chest CT. *Radiology* 2020: 200905. https://doi.org/10.1148/radiol.2020200905.
58. Ebrahimian M, Behnam B, Ghayebi N, Sobhrakhshankhah E. ChatGPT in Iranian medical licensing examination: Evaluating the diagnostic accuracy and decision-making capabilities of an AI-based model. *BMJ Health Care Inform* 2023; 30(1): e100815. https://doi.org/10.1136/bmjhci-2023-100815.
59. McKinney SM, Sieniek M, Godbole V, et al. International evaluation of an AI system for breast cancer screening. *Nature* 2020; 577(7788): 89–94. https://doi.org/10.1038/s41586-019-1799-6.
60. Han R, Acosta JN, Shakeri Z, et al. Randomised controlled trials evaluating artificial intelligence in clinical practice: A scoping review. *Lancet Digit Health* 2024; 6(5): e367–e373. https://doi.org/10.1016/S2589-7500(24)00047-5.
61. Sujan M, Furniss D, Grundy K, et al. Human factors challenges for the safe use of artificial intelligence in patient care. *BMJ Health Care Inform* 2019; 26(1): e100081. https://doi.org/10.1136/bmjhci-2019-100081.
62. Sujan MA, White S, Habli I, Reynolds N. Stakeholder perceptions of the safety and assurance of artificial intelligence in healthcare. *Saf Sci* 2022; 155: 105870. https://doi.org/10.1016/j.ssci.2022.105870.
63. Sujan M, Baber C, Salmon P, Pool R, Chozos N. Human Factors and Ergonomics in Healthcare AI. Wootton Waven: Chartered Institute of Ergonomics and Human Factors, 2021. https://bit.ly/AIinHealthcareWP (accessed 10 January 2026).
64. Sujan M, Pool R, Salmon P. Eight human factors and ergonomics principles for healthcare artificial intelligence. *BMJ Health Care Inform* 2022; 29(1): e100516. https://doi.org/10.1136/bmjhci-2021-100516.
65. Hignett S, Bowie P. Why is the NHS still harming patients? Taking a professional approach to patient safety for COVID-19 and beyond. *Sci Parliament* 2020; 76(3): 14–16.

66. Hignett S, Cook S, Maguire M, Taylor E. Human factors and ergonomics throughout the lifespan. In Kopec D, ed. *Health and Wellbeing for Interior Architecture*. New York: Routledge, 2017.
67. Hignett S, Lu J. Space to care and treat safely in acute hospitals: Recommendations from 1866 to 2008. *Appl Ergon* 2010; 41(5): 666–673. https://doi.org/10.1016/j.apergo.2009.12.010.
68. Hignett S, Lu J, Fray M. Two case studies using mock-ups for planning adult and neonatal intensive care facilities. *J Healthc Eng* 2010; 1(3): 399–414. https://doi.org/10.1260/2040-2295.1.3.399.
69. Sarker SK, Chang A, Albrani T, Vincent C. Constructing hierarchical task analysis in surgery. *Surg Endosc* 2008; 22(1): 107–111. https://doi.org/10.1007/s00464-007-9380-z.
70. Hignett S. Technology and building design: Initiatives to reduce inpatient falls among the elderly. *HERD* 2010; 3(4): 93–105. https://doi.org/10.1177/193758671000300408.
71. Hignett S, Lu J. Evaluation of critical care space requirements for three frequent and high-risk tasks. *Crit Care Nurs Clin North Am* 2007; 19(2): 167–175. https://doi.org/10.1016/j.ccell.2007.02.004.
72. Kwok Y-t, Lam M-s. Using human factors and ergonomics principles to prevent inpatient falls. *BMJ Open Qual* 2022; 11(1): e001696. https://doi.org/10.1136/bmjoq-2021-001696.
73. MohammadiGorji S, Joseph A, Mihandoust S, et al. Anesthesia workspaces for safe medication practices: Design guidelines. *HERD* 2024; 17(1): 64–83. https://doi.org/10.1177/19375867231190646.
74. Peek N, Sujan M, Scott P. Digital health and care: Emerging from pandemic times. *BMJ Health Care Inform* 2023; 30(1): e100861. https://doi.org/10.1136/bmjhci-2023-100861.
75. Lee AC, Cousens S, Wall SN, et al. Neonatal resuscitation and immediate newborn assessment and stimulation for the prevention of neonatal deaths: A systematic review, meta-analysis and Delphi estimation of mortality effect. *BMC Public Health* 2011; 11(S3): S12. https://doi.org/10.1186/1471-2458-11-S3-S12.
76. Liberati EG, Tarrant C, Willars J, et al. Seven features of safety in maternity units: A framework based on multisite ethnography and stakeholder consultation. *BMJ Qual Saf* 2021; 30(6): 444–456. https://doi.org/10.1136/bmjqs-2020-010988.
77. Pickup L, Lang A, Shipley L, et al. Development of a clinical interface for a Novel newborn resuscitation device: Human factors approach to understanding cognitive user requirements. *JMIR Hum Factors* 2019; 6(2): e12055. https://doi.org/10.2196/12055.

78. Militello LG, Hutton RJB. Applied cognitive task analysis (ACTA): A practitioner's toolkit for understanding cognitive task demands. *Ergonomics* 1998; 41(11): 1618–1641. https://doi.org/10.1080/001401398186108.
79. Carman E-M, Johnson M, Miles G. Human factors and procurement: Lessons learnt from a high-value procurement exercise. In Balfe, N, Charles, R, Golightly, D, eds. *Ergonomics and Human Factors*. Warwickshire: Chartered Institute for Ergonomics and Human Factors; 2023.
80. Habli I, White S, Sujan M, Harrison S, Ugarte M. What is the safety case for health IT? A study of assurance practices in England. *Saf Sci* 2018; 110: 324–335. https://doi.org/10.1016/j.ssci.2018.09.001.
81. Card AJ. Patient safety 2.0: Slaying dragons, not just investigating them. *J Patient Saf* 2023; 19(6): 394–395. https://doi.org/10.1097/PTS.0000000000001140.
82. Hignett S, Jones EL, Miller D, et al. Human factors and ergonomics and quality improvement science: Integrating approaches for safety in healthcare. *BMJ Qual Saf* 2015; 24(4): 250. https://doi.org/10.1136/bmjqs-2014-003623.
83. Carayon P, Wetterneck TB, Rivera-Rodriguez AJ, et al. Human factors systems approach to healthcare quality and patient safety. *Appl Ergon* 2014; 45(1): 14–25. https://doi.org/10.1016/j.apergo.2013.04.023.
84. Joint Commission. People, processes, health IT and accurate patient identification. Quick Safety Issue. 45. The Joint Commission, 2018. https://digitalassets.jointcommission.org/api/public/content/2dc4cad7bdc34451b85a2be5431f09ef (accessed 10 January 2026).
85. Care Quality Commission. Ionising Radiation (Medical Exposure) Regulations Annual Report 2023/24. 2024. www.cqc.org.uk/publications/irmer-annual-report/2023-2024/summary#:~:text=From%201%20April%202023%20to,%2C%20an%20increase%20of%2013%25 (accessed 10 January 2026).
86. Woodward M, Nayak R, McCulloch P. Radiography as a sociotechnical system – Improving patient identification with a multi-level human factors approach. *Saf Sci* 2022; 150: 105679. https://doi.org/10.1016/j.ssci.2022.105679.
87. Carayon P, Hundt AS, Karsh B, et al. Work system design for patient safety: The SEIPS model. *BMJ Qual Saf* 2006; 15(suppl 1): i50–i58. https://doi.org/10.1136/qshc.2005.015842.
88. DeRosier J, Stalhandske E, Bagian JP, Nudell T. Using health care failure mode and effect analysis: The VA national center for patient safety's

prospective risk analysis system. *Jt Comm J Qual Improv* 2002; 28(5): 248–67. https://doi.org/10.1016/s1070-3241(02)28025-6.

89. Sujan M, Crumpton E, Finch V, Combes J. From vision to reality: How human factors can inform the design of cardiac diagnostic services in community settings. *Hum Factors Healthc* 2024; 5: 100075. https://doi.org/10.1016/j.hfh.2024.100075.
90. Holden RJ, Carayon P. SEIPS 101 and seven simple SEIPS tools. *BMJ Qual Saf* 2021; 30: 901–910. https://doi.org/10.1136/bmjqs-2020-012538.
91. National Advisory Group on the Safety of Patients in England. *A Promise to Learn – A Commitment to Act*. London: Department of Health, 2013. https://assets.publishing.service.gov.uk/media/5a7cc74540f0b6629523bc31/Berwick_Report.pdf (accessed 10th January 2026).
92. Stanton NA, Margaryan A, Littlejohn A. Editorial: Learning from incidents. *Saf Sci* 2017; 99: 1–4. https://doi.org/10.1016/j.ssci.2017.07.011.
93. Hollnagel E, Sujan M, Braithwaite J. Resilient health care – Making steady progress. *Saf Sci* 2019; 120: 781–782. https://doi.org/10.1016/j.ssci.2019.07.029.
94. Rasmussen J. Risk management in a dynamic society: A modelling problem. *Saf Sci* 1997; 27(2–3): 183–213. https://doi.org/10.1016/S0925-7535(97)00052-0.
95. Svendung I, Rasmussen J. Graphic representation of accident scenarios: Mapping system structure and causation of accidents. *Saf Sci* 2002; 40(5): 397–417. https://doi.org/10.1016/S0925-7535(00)00036-9.
96. Salmon PM, King B, Hulme A, et al. Toward the translation of systems thinking methods in patient safety practice: Assessing the validity of Net-HARMS and AcciMap. *Saf Sci* 2023; 159. https://doi.org/10.1016/j.ssci.2022.106003.
97. Salmon P, Coventon L, Read G. Understanding and preventing work-related violence in hospital settings: A systems thinking approach. Centre for Human Factors and Sociotechnical Systems University of the Sunshine Coast, 2021. www.safework.nsw.gov.au/__data/assets/pdf_file/0006/964716/understanding-and-preventing-work-related-violence-in-hospital-settings-a-systems-thinking-approach.pdf (accessed 10 January 2026).
98. Rae AJ, Provan DJ, Weber DE, Dekker SW. Safety clutter: The accumulation and persistence of 'safety' work that does not contribute to operational safety. *Policy and Pract Health Saf* 2018; 16(2): 194–211. https://doi.org/10.1080/14773996.2018.1491147.
99. Goode N, Read GJM, Van Mulken MRH, Clacy A, Salmon PM. Designing system reforms: Using a systems approach to translate incident analyses

into prevention strategies. *Front Psychol* 2016; 7: 1974. https://doi.org/10.3389/fpsyg.2016.01974.

100. Safework. Preventing work-related violence systems thinking in incident investigations guide. New South Wales Government; 2022. www.safework.nsw.gov.au/__data/assets/pdf_file/0017/1210355/systems-thinking-for-preventing-work-related-violence-in-hospitals.pdf (accessed 10 January 2026).
101. Sujan MA, Huang H, Braithwaite J. Learning from incidents in health care: Critique from a safety-II perspective. *Saf Sci* 2017; 99: 115–121. https://doi.org/10.1016/j.ssci.2016.08.005.
102. Health Services Safety Investigations Body. Investigation report: COVID-19 transmission in hospitals – Management of the risk (a prospective safety investigation). 2020/10/29/ 2020. www.hssib.org.uk/patient-safety-investigations/covid-19-transmission-in-hospitals-management-of-the-risk/investigation-report/#executive-summary (accessed 10 January 2026).
103. Wilson JR. Fundamentals of systems ergonomics/human factors. *Appl Ergon* 2014; 45(1): 5–13. https://doi.org/10.1016/j.apergo.2013.03.021.
104. Stanton N, Salmon PM, Rafferty LA, et al. *Human Factors Methods: A Practical Guide for Engineering and Design*. Ashgate; 2013.
105. Waterson P. A critical review of the systems approach within patient safety research. *Ergonomics* 2009; 52(10): 1185–1195. https://doi.org/10.1080/00140130903042782.
106. Dekker S. *Safety Differently*. CRC Press: London; 2014.
107. Catchpole K, Bowie P, Fouquet S, Rivera J, Hignett S. Frontiers in human factors: Embedding specialists in multi-disciplinary efforts to improve healthcare. *Int J Qual Health Care* 2021; 33(Supplement_1): 13–18. https://doi.org/10.1093/intqhc/mzaa108.
108. Rae A, Provan D, Aboelssaad H, Alexander R. A manifesto for Reality-based Safety Science. *Saf Sci* 2020; 126: 104654. https://doi.org/10.1016/j.ssci.2020.104654.
109. Sujan MA, Habli I, Kelly TP, Pozzi S, Johnson CW. Should healthcare providers do safety cases? Lessons from a cross-industry review of safety case practices. *Saf Sci* 2016; 84: 181–189. https://doi.org/10.1016/j.ssci.2015.12.021.
110. Sujan M, Pickup L, de Vos MS, et al. Operationalising FRAM in healthcare: A critical reflection on practice. *Saf Sci* 2023; 158: 105994. https://doi.org/10.1016/j.ssci.2022.105994.
111. Dixon-Woods M, Martin GP. Does quality improvement improve quality? *Future Hosp J* 2016; 3(3): 191–194. https://doi.org/10.7861/futurehosp.3-3-191.

112. Skivington K, Matthews L, Simpson SA, et al. A new framework for developing and evaluating complex interventions: Update of Medical Research Council guidance. *BMJ* 2021; 374: n2061. https://doi.org/10.1136/bmj.n2061.
113. Pawson R, Tilley N. *Realistic Evaluation*. London: Sage; 1997.
114. Dixon-Woods M, Bosk CL, Aveling EL, Goeschel CA, Pronovost PJ. Explaining Michigan: Developing an ex post theory of a quality improvement program. *Milbank Q* 2011; 89(2): 167–205. https://doi.org/10.1111/j.1468-0009.2011.00625.x.
115. May C, Finch T. Implementing, embedding, and integrating practices: An outline of normalization process theory. *Sociology* 2009; 43(3): 535–554. https://doi.org/10.1177/0038038509103208.
116. Dixon-Woods M. How to improve healthcare improvement – an essay by Mary Dixon-Woods. *BMJ* 2019; 367: l5514. https://doi.org/10.1136/bmj.l5514.
117. Eurocontrol. A Business Case for Human Factors Investment. https://skybrary.aero/bookshelf/human-factors-module-business-case-human-factors-investment-0 (accessed 10 January 2026).
118. Sujan M, Pickup L, Vosper H, Catchpole K. *Human Factors and Ergonomics in Health and Social Care: An Applied Approach*. Bridgwater: Class Professional; 2025.
119. Wilson JR, Sharples S. *Evaluation of Human Work*: CRC Press; 2015.

Cambridge Elements

Improving Quality and Safety in Healthcare

Gemma Petley

THIS Institute (The Healthcare Improvement Studies Institute)

Gemma is Senior Communications and Editorial Manager at THIS Institute, responsible for overseeing the production and maximising the impact of the series.

Claire Dipple

THIS Institute (The Healthcare Improvement Studies Institute)

Claire is Editorial Project Manager at THIS Institute, responsible for editing and projectmanaging the series.

About the Series

The past decade has seen enormous growth in both activity and research on improvement in healthcare. This series offers a comprehensive and authoritative set of overviews of the different improvement approaches available, exploring the thinking behind them, examining evidence for each approach, and identifying areas of debate.

Cambridge Elements

Improving Quality and Safety in Healthcare

Elements in the Series

Simulation as an Improvement Technique
Victoria Brazil, Eve Purdy, and Komal Bajaj

Workplace Conditions
Jill Maben, Jane Ball, and Amy C. Edmondson

Governance and Leadership
Naomi J. Fulop and Angus I. G. Ramsay

Health Economics
Andrew Street and Nils Gutacker

Approaches to Spread, Scale-Up, and Sustainability
Chrysanthi Papoutsi, Trisha Greenhalgh, and Sonja Marjanovic

Statistical Process Control
Mohammed Amin Mohammed

Values and Ethics
Alan Cribb, Vikki Entwistle, and Polly Mitchell

Design Creativity
Gyuchan Thomas Jun, Sue Hignett and P. John Clarkson

Supply Chain Management
Sharon J. Williams

Measurement for Improvement
Alene Toulany and Kaveh G. Shojania

Learning Health Systems
Thomas Foley and Leora I. Horwitz

Clinical Microsystems and Team Coaching
Steve Harrison, Rachael Finn and Marjorie M. Godfrey

Audit, Feedback, and Behaviour Change
Noah Ivers and Robbie Foy

Human Factors and Ergonomics
Mark Sujan and Laura Pickup

A full series listing is available at: www.cambridge.org/IQ